SMOOTHIE RECIPES

Best Strawberry Smoothie Cookbook Ever for Beginners

(Simple, Easy and Very Healthy Smoothie Recipes Green Smoothies)

Emmett Ulrich

Published by Alex Howard

© **Emmett Ulrich**

All Rights Reserved

Smoothie Recipes: Best Strawberry Smoothie Cookbook Ever for Beginners (Simple, Easy and Very Healthy Smoothie Recipes Green Smoothies)

ISBN 978-1-990169-80-9

All rights reserved. No part of this guide may be reproduced in any form without permission in writing from the publisher except in the case of brief quotations embodied in critical articles or reviews.

Legal & Disclaimer

The information contained in this book is not designed to replace or take the place of any form of medicine or professional medical advice. The information in this book has been provided for educational and entertainment purposes only.

The information contained in this book has been compiled from sources deemed reliable, and it is accurate to the best of the Author's knowledge; however, the Author cannot guarantee its accuracy and validity and cannot be held liable for any errors or omissions. Changes are periodically made to this book. You must consult your doctor or get professional medical advice before using any of the suggested remedies, techniques, or information in this book.

Table of contents

Part 1 1

Introduction 2

Chapter 1: Introduction To Green Smoothie And Its Amazing Benefits 4

Chapter 2: Smoothie Drinks And Their Effects On Health 12

Chapter 3: 20 Step Goal To Challenge Your Body For Weight Loss 19

Chapter 4: Best Healthy Detox Smoothie Recipes.......................24

Recipe No.1: Green Peachy Protein Smoothie 25

Recipe No. 2: Detox Spring Smoothie..26

Recipe No. 3: Kale Protein Smoothie...27

Recipe No. 4: Green Happy Monster...28

Recipe No 5: Spinach Orange Smoothie.......................................29

Recipe No. 6: Pear Green Protein Smoothie Recipe 30

Recipe No. 7: Orange Kale Green Juice Recipe 31

Recipe No. 8: Ginger-Orange Green Smoothie Recipe.............32

Recipe No. 9: Green Skin Cleanser 33

Recipe No. 10: Tropical Green Smoothie.....................................34

Recipe No.11: Blueberry Mint Green Smoothie 35

Recipe No. 12: Spring Detox Smoothie...36

Chapter 5: Success Stories Of People Benefiting From Smoothie Detox Drinks 37

Chapter 6: Smoothie Recipes 43

Apples And Cream Smoothie 43

Apple Carrot Quencher 44

Avocado Avalanche 45

Avocado Banana Berry Smoothie 46

Banana Blueberry Smoothie 47

Banana Orange Twist 48

Banana Split Smoothie 49

Berry Blue Smoothie 50

Blackberry Smoothie 51

Blueberry Maple Smoothie 52

Cappuccino Smoothie 53

Cherry Vanilla Smoothie 54

Chocolate Banana Smoothie 55

Double Apple Smoothie 56

Frozen Fruit Smoothie 57

Fruit Salad Smoothie 58

Guava Smoothie 59

Hawaiian Silk Smoothie 60

Honey Raspberry Smoothie 61

Kiwi Cooler 62

Lemon Lime Smoothie 63

Lemonade Sweet Tart Smoothie 64

Mango Smoothie 65

Mexican Smoothie 66

Orange Pineapple Smoothie 67

Organic Smoothie 68

Papaya Smoothie 69

Peaches And Dreams Smoothie 70

Peanut Butter Smoothie 71

Peanut Butter Sundae Smoothie 72

Peppermint Smoothie 73

Pina Banana Smoothie 74

Pina Colada Smoothie 75

Pineapple Papaya Smoothie 76

Pink Smoothie Deluxe 77

Purple Passion Smoothie 78

Rainbow Smoothie 79

Raspberry Orange Smoothie 80

Raspberry Watermelon Smoothie 81

Smoothie Power Shake 82

Strawberry Banana Smoothie 83

Strawberry Blueberry Smoothie 84

Strawberry Kiwi Smoothie 85

Strawberry Lemonade Smoothie 86

Strawberry Raspberry Smoothie 87

Strawberry Sunrise Smoothie 88

Tangerine Dreams Smoothie 89

Tropical Fling Smoothie 90

Wacky Watermelon Smoothie 91

Zippy Pineapple Carrot Smoothie 92

Conclusion 93

Part 2 94

Introduction 95

Coconut & Watermelon Smoothie 121

Avocado Smoothie 122

Cabbage With Berry Smoothie 123

Green Leaf Smoothie 124

Simple Green Protein Smoothie 125

Vanilla Yogurt Smoothie 126

Carrot Smoothie 127

Grapefruit Smoothie 128

Papaya Smoothie 129

Almond Smoothie 130

Celery & Tomato Smoothie 131

Beet Green Smoothie 132

Zucchini Smoothie 133

Green Aloe Juice	134
Anti Aging Smoothie	135
Green Smoothie	136
Dr. Oz's Green Smoothie	137
Healthy Skin Smoothie	138
Antioxidant Smoothie	139
Berry Medley Smoothie	140
Vitamin C Smoothie	141
Healthy Hair Smoothie	142
Super Detox Green Smoothie	143
Healthy Herb Smoothie	144
Ginger Detox Smoothies	145
Smoothies Recipes	146
Strawberry Kale Smoothie	146
Apple Orange Smoothie	147
Kale Banana Smoothie	148
Cucumber Kale Smoothie	149
Berry Spinach Smoothie	150
Pineapple Mango Smoothie	151
Peach Kale Smoothie	153
Avocado Banana Smoothie	154
Grape Banana Smoothie	155
Pear Spinach Smoothie	156

Berry Smoothie	157
Gingery Kale Smoothie	158
Kale Banana Smoothie	159
Chard Mango Smoothie	160
Grape Wheat Grass Smoothie	161
Watermelon Lettuce Smoothie	162
Pomegranate Berry	163
Tropical Smoothie	164
Tofu Strawberry Smoothie	165
Peach Arugula Smoothie	166
Spiced Orange Smoothie	167
Banana Smoothie	168
Fruity Smoothie	169
Banana Berry Smoothie	170
Easy Strawberry Lemonade	171
Grab It And Go Shake!	172
Orange Creamsicle Shake	173
Strawberry Banana Smoothie	174
Peppermint Patty Shake	175
Chocolate Mint Shake	176
Grapefruit Surprise Shake	177
Restaurant Style Italian Soda	178
Root Beer Float	179

Blueberry Smoothie 180

Iced Coffee Shake 181

Iced Mocha Shake 182

Maple Nut Shake... 183

Almond Joy Shake 184

Banana Blast Smoothie 185

Chocolate Covered Banana Smoothie 186

Chocolate Covered Cherries Smoothie 187

Raspberry Smoothie................... **Error! Bookmark not defined.**

Cinnamon Roll Protein Shake **Error! Bookmark not defined.**

Conclusion... 188

Part 1

Introduction

Are you overweight? Do you find yourself stuck in the diet plans that never seem to work? Have you compromised on your health while trying to lose your weight? Are you spending more on your diet than on your nutrition? Do you often find yourself cheating on your diet plan? Do you wish to be healthy again? If yes then it is time to relax because this book brings you the kind of diet plan that you will never ever cheat on as it comes with simple, cheap and easy way to lose weight without losing your health. The diet plan discussed in this book consists of simple raw fruits and vegetables that must be blended together to give you a likeable taste and a cup full of nutrients. All that your belly needs!

The book is written with the intention to help you maintain a balance between your diet and your health so that you can maximize the benefits out of this 'losing the weight' mission. Those who follow diet plans need to realize that either under or overweight or even just the right weight, there is no use of any weight without health. Therefore, choosing a diet plan should always be based on the benefits it does to your overall health. Green detox smoothies serve all the above mentioned purposes though following the diet plan made out of it requires persistence and patience but once you see the results, your lifestyle will forever be changed and for good.

Chapter 1: Introduction To Green Smoothie And Its Amazing Benefits

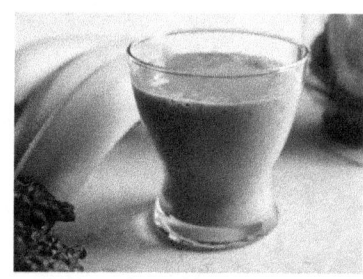

Wonder if you could brew a magic potion that can recharge you, clear your system from the unwanted toxins and is ready in less than 13 minutes. Sounds great, right? Green smoothies are tasty, healthy, full of nutrients and easy to make.

You won't experience the gross flavor of raw veggies and your palate would not find it tasteless. When smoothies are made with veggies and mixed with the fruits they give you the kind of delight that you would desire every time. The smoothies are full of green food, rich in fibers which slow down the process of absorption of fruit sugars thus, provide you with just the appropriate amount of energy and nutrition that your body really needs and loves.

Rich in nutrients:

If you're worried and really concerned that you're not getting enough nutrients required by your body, you should start taking green smoothies on daily basis. The more green smoothies you consume; the more amino acid is produced which in turn is used to synthesize proteins in your body.

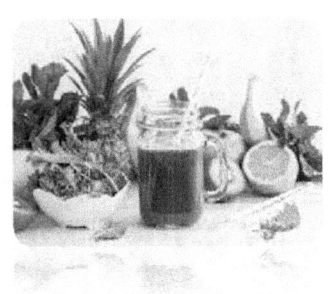

Healthy way of eating raw food:

Intake of green smoothies is the gateway to a healthy food addiction. Though it takes time to make them a regular part of your life but the short term results are pretty convincing and motivating. It gives your skin a fresh glow which makes you look younger and active. Who does not like to look good?

Green smoothies are detoxifiers:

Green smoothies play a vital role in detoxifying the body and carry with them countless health benefits. These detoxifying smoothies may include a blend of spinach, parsley, lettuce, and collard greens. For more delicious green smoothie drinks you can also add kale, dandelion greens, watercress. Moreover, you can improve its taste by adding bananas, mango, apple, avocado and pears.

Following is a list of benefits that green smoothies can provide, if you take them on a daily basis:

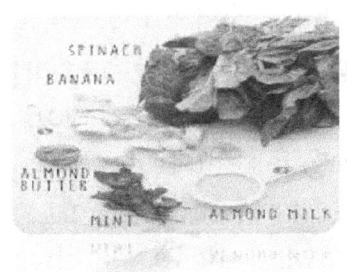

1. **Nourishment**: Green smoothies provide you with the right nutrients. The precursors of vitamins in your body comes from the vegetables and the fruits therefore, consuming them meets your nutritional demands. Though, most vegetables and fruits are high in vitamins A and C, some others like avocado gives you high amounts of potassium and magnesium which are also vital for your body.

2. **Smoothies are healthier than juice:** Green smoothies are much healthier and more beneficial to the body than the juices extracted from vegetables and fruits because 'juicing' leaves you with the minerals and the vitamins only whereas, smoothies provide you the fiber as well which is beneficial to your body in several ways.
3. **Easy way to eat veggies:** Green smoothies are easy way to eat veggies without even consciously recognizing it. While most people like fruits and many of them have trouble eating the veggies because of its taste, green smoothies are a perfect way to sweeten the odd taste of the green food because of the added fruits.
4. **Time saving:** Green smoothies are quick and easy to make. The only equipment you need is a blender and some veggies and fruits.
5. **Affordable:** Homemade green smoothies are easy to make and are cheap. Purchasing smoothies can cost you as much as $5 a glass. At home, you can make it by adding fruits and vegetables, which won't cost you more than a few cents. Drinking one glass every day will provide you with all the vitamins your body requires and the good point is, it is cheaper than buying multivitamins.

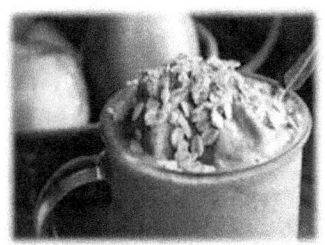

6. **Give kids a new taste:** Green smoothies can be a best way to convince your kids to eat their vegetables in a more easy-to-take-in way because they would not even complain about the usual odd taste of the vegetables. For making it easier on the kids, start with a higher proportion of the fruits rather than the vegetables.

7. **Long lasting energy:** Green smoothies will give you a long lasting source of energy. When you eat fruits they only provide momentary energy due to high levels of sugars they contain but the sugars are quickly metabolized in the body whereas, in the form of smoothies, they have a balanced sugar content and the fibers slow down the sugar consumption as a result you remain active for longer.
8. **Full meal:** Green smoothies are heavy in nutrients and low in calories and contain high amounts of water and fiber which is required by your body. If you're on a diet or trying to lose weight, the best way to fight your cravings is to use the green smoothies. You will stick longer to your plan!
9. **Easy digestion:** Green smoothies are quickly digested because they're already blended and liquefied. People suffering from indigestion problem after eating meals should try green smoothies. It will help them with their digestion process.

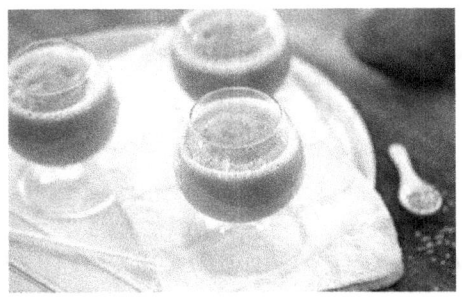

10. **Keep the body hydrated**: Green smoothies will keep the body hydrated. Our body requires 8 glasses of water daily but most of us do not even drink half of the amount required. The main reason is most of the people don't like the taste of the ordinary water. Smoothies will not only give you better taste but will also act as a supplement to water the requirement.

Chapter 2: Smoothie Drinks And Their Effects On Health

Let's suppose you are trying to make a green smoothie. You reach your refrigerator, grab some fruits and veggies and take the yoghurt and milk bottle along with some ice cubes. Next, you switch on the blender and mix all the stuff up and voila! It's ready! Veggies usually are not served in the form of juices as blending is an easy way to get the maximum benefits out of it.

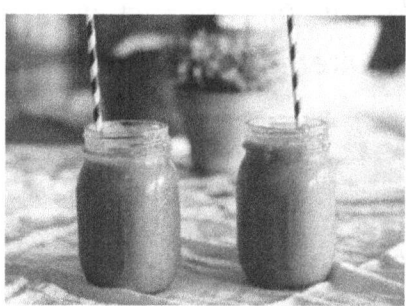

Add some more greens in smoothies:

Healthy food aids your immune system to help you defeat the bad guys in your body. If you take 60 to 80% of green smoothies in your diet then you have it all. Also, know that the greens in your bowl will not give you a bad taste in mouth because you can always add fruits, milk or yoghurt for balancing the taste according to your preference. An easy way to get started is to use spinach and romaine. After that you can try some collard, kale, lettuce, cucumber and some green herbs in small quantity. In case, you don't like the taste of the bitter greens you can always change your proportions.

Swiss chard smoothie benefits:

Swiss chard has soft leaves and adds a good flavor to your smoothies. You can also mix it with sour or tart fruit. 1 cup of Swiss chard smoothie has less than 10 calories and gives your body the full dose of potassium, magnesium and calcium. It is also rich in vitamin A, C and K to support your immune system. Furthermore, it gives you strong vision and strength to your bones and also regulates the blood flow in the body.

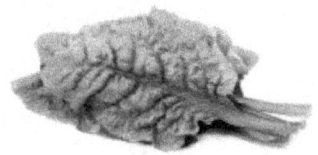

Spinach smoothie benefits:

Commonly the spinach's green leaves are used in smoothies. It has soft texture and mild flavor which is a perfect match for sweet and sour smoothies. A cup of it has less than 10 calories. It is rich in magnesium, calcium and potassium. It also provides your body some good amount of vitamins A, C and K.

Dandelion greens benefits:

Dandelion green works as a cleansing agent, it is rich in phosphorous, magnesium, potassium and calcium along with vitamins A and K. It positively effects the function of kidney, liver and gallbladder. Dandelion is a bit bitter in taste so better keep it in less quantity but you can slowly increase the amount according to your taste and mood. You can also mix it with strong flavored fruits like orange, pineapple and banana to minimize the taste of the bitterness.

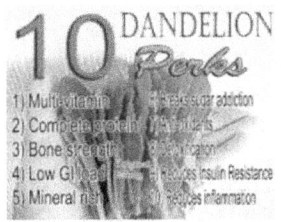

Avocado

Avocado is also another type of green veggie but it's not in the form of leaves. It is a great source of protein and monounsaturated fat that protects the heart and fight against the diseases. It also makes you feel full for a long time. It is high in folate, potassium, phosphorus, calcium, magnesium and contain high levels of vitamin C and fiber.

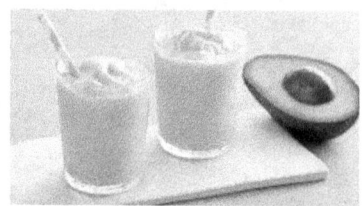

Following are some of the long term healthy effects of the green veggies:

Improve and build muscle: It helps the muscles to rebuild and recover after an injury or a heavy work out.

Personal health goals: Smoothies help you to stick to your diet goals.

Beauty enhancer: Green vegetable are the good for the hair, skin and nails. They supply the adequate amount of minerals and vitamins required for the healthier and glowing body structure.

Strengthen immune system: "Health is wealth" and sickness leads to you many physical and social problems. To overcome diseases, improving immune system and getting an overall healthy life green smoothies work just fine.

Sound and peaceful sleep: It also helps to improve your sleep cycle.

Meal flexibility: Smoothies are what you can consume easily, you don't need a lot of time to prepare them. If you don't have time for breakfast, lunch or dinner just grab a smoothie and give your body a boost of energy.

Brain boost: Brain when provided with the right nutrients can do wonders. Green smoothies can improve your mental activity like clarity, memory and focus. So, shake hand with green smoothies and say goodbye to the brain fog.

Happiness: When your belly is filled and the nutrients are being provided properly to your body and brain, you feel active and live and a result a sense of calm and well-being prevails over you.

Chapter 3: 20 Step Goal To Challenge Your Body For Weight Loss

If you want to get in shape then get ready for a 30 days challenge to lose the extra fat on your body. Accept the challenge and follow the following steps:

1. **Forget the shame and blame:** Don't take things in life very personally or put pressure on yourself. You are your own master and you have the authority to decide how you want to look like. Forget about the society, follow your heart.
2. **Set Goals:** Goal setting is very important in life for anything and when you decide to lose weight, remember that it will take time, it is a long term goal with baby steps. You have to be more specific, measurable of your time and the challenge you are taking and must achieve the small step first to eventually start running.
3. **Ditch the Sugar:** High intake of sugar can lead to many problems like heart disease and weight gain so, say good bye to the sugar and welcome honey in your life. Sacrifice is the rule!
4. **Avoid Carbs:** Nutritionists suggest you should take more fiber in your diet rather than carbohydrates as fibers help you in losing weight.
5. **Forget about the soft drinks:** Soft drinks are full of sugar. Say no to them

6. **Treat yourself:** Giving yourself a little treat will motivate you to achieve your goal more quickly. The treat should be your favorite snack, given once each week during the weight loss.
7. **Keep grains in check:** Grain should be added up in the small meal because they fill your tummy and are low in calories. Whole grains should be serving in your plan in 3 different days.
8. **Eat only when feel hungry:** People usually eat when they are sad or depressed or bored. Stop yourself from such kind of munching. Eat only when you are hungry.

9. **Go for a walk:** You must add walk in your plan. Start form 30 minutes and gradually increase it to 2 hours.
10. **Never skip breakfast:** Start your day with good and healthy diet which is full of fiber and protein.
11. **Meal preparation:** The more time you spend in the kitchen the more craving you will feel to eat. Use quick meals and avoid unnecessary visits to the kitchen.
12. **Keep a food journal:** Make the habit of keeping a food journal during the challenge so you know what are you eating and what are you going to eat. Make a list and of healthy products which are full of protein like boil egg and rich in fiber like green smoothies. Write on the daily basis at the start of the day and at the end of the day. Monitor your hunger.
13. **Add protein intake:** While losing weight it is suggested to intake more protein in your diet. You can take it in the form of nuts.
14. **Put veggies or fruit on every plate:** Veggies and fruit are a must in the diet plan. They can be in the raw form or in the boil or you can add smoothies.
15. **Know your healthy fats:** Healthy fats are olive oil, nuts and avocados.
16. **Eliminate your distractions:** According to the researches while eating if you are distracted, you can consume high amount of calories which is not

good for your goal. So, turn of the TV or smart phone.
17. **Check weight machine:** You should note down your weight daily and look how many numbers have fallen or gone up and in how many days. This will motivate you to lose weight and put more effort.

18. **Sleep 7+ hours:**. Lack of sleep could be a havoc on your weight loss goal. Hormones that control hunger will send more signal to the brain to get hungry.
19. **Work out is essential like nutrient:** Make a daily routine to do few minute workout. Work out does not only helps your body to lose some calorie but also it helps your body to get in good shape and improve your posture.
20. **Yoga:** Add yoga to your goal. It relaxes your mind and body and make it ready to achieve your goals.

Chapter 4: Best Healthy Detox Smoothie Recipes

Recipe No.1: Green Peachy Protein Smoothie

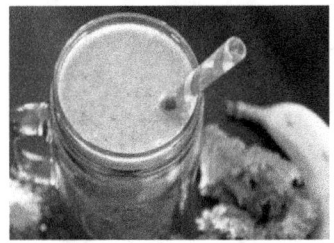

Preparation time: 5 minutes

Servings: 2 pals or you can take two times a day.

Ingredients:

2 spoon of vanilla essence

Add one up of almond milk it should unsweetened

Pour 1 cup of peaches that you can freeze for one hour before using it.

Add 1/2 cup of pineapple

2 ½ pealed banana

Add 2 cups of kale

Add1 tbsp. of ground flaxseed.

Directions:

Put all the ingredients into the blender and blend it for 3 to 4 minutes until you get a good creamy texture.

Recipe No. 2: Detox Spring Smoothie

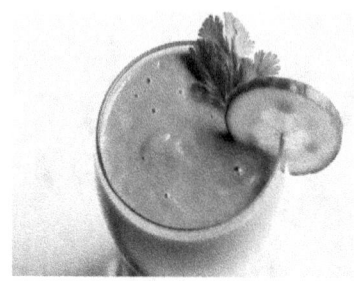

This smoothie is full of natural detoxifying fruits and veggies that help you feel great.

Preparation time: Hardly 5 minutes

You can serve: 1 glass

Ingredients:

- Add 1 cup of chilled green tea
- Add 1 cup of cilantro.
- Add 1 cup of Organic baby kale.
- Add 1 cup of fresh cucumber
- Add 1 cup juicy pineapple
- Squeeze 1 lemon juice.
- Add 1 tbsp. of fresh grated ginger
- Add ½ slice of avocado

Directions:

Add every ingredient in the blender. Blend these ingredients till you get a smooth texture like a cream.

Recipe No. 3: Kale Protein Smoothie

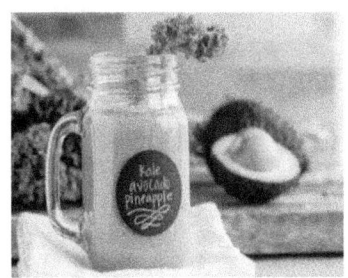

Preparation time: 7 minutes

Servings: 3 glass of smoothies

Ingredients you want for this smoothie:

- Pour 2/3 cup of vanilla almond milk but it should be unsweetened.
- Add 2 large kale
- Add 1/3 chunks of pineapple
- Add 1/2 slice avocado
- 1 tsp protein powder
- 1 cup of ice

Directions:

Take a blender and add every ingredient in this blender.

Recipe No. 4: Green Happy Monster

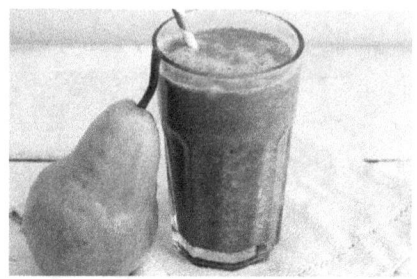

Time required: 10 Minutes

Servings: 2 glass of smoothies

Ingredients for blending:
- Pour 1 glass of coconut water
- Pour 1/3 glass of coconut milk
- Add 1 tbsp. of agave syrup
- Squeeze juice of half lime
- Add 1 peeled pear
- Add 2 cup of spinach
- Add 2 cup of kale

Directions:

Take all ingredients and blend them together in the blender to get a smooth and yummy creamy smoothie.

Recipe No 5: Spinach Orange Smoothie

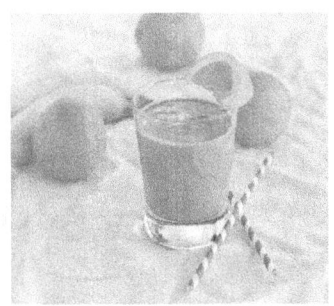

Preparation time: 5 minutes

Servings: 2 glass.

Ingredients:

- Add 1 peeled orange.
- Add 1/2 peeled banana, peeled
- Add 1 cup of spinach
- Add 1/4 cup of coconut water or adjust with the paste.
- 1 tablespoon of hemp seed if you like it.

Directions:

Add all the ingredients in the blender. Blend these ingredients to get a smooth texture like a cream.

Recipe No. 6: Pear Green Protein Smoothie Recipe

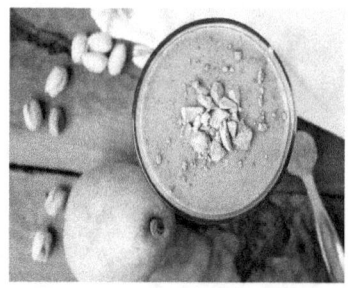

Time for preparation: 5 - 7 minutes

Servings: 1 glass

Ingredients to be added:

Add 1 tsp of vanilla

Add 1 cup of almond milk

Add 1 cup of spinach

Add 1 peeled pear

Add 1/2 tsp of matcha tea powder

Directions:

Blend every ingredient in the blender. Blend these ingredients to get a smooth and creamy texture.

Recipe No. 7: Orange Kale Green Juice Recipe

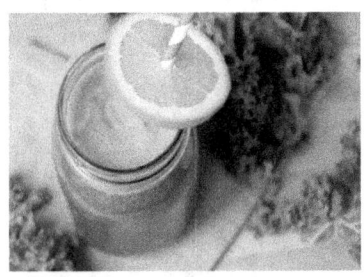

Time for preparation: 8 minutes

Serving: 1 glass

Ingredients needed:

- Add 1 packet of vanilla flavor
- Pour 1 cup of water in the blender
- Add 1 raw green kale
- Add 1 Peeled large orange
- Half tsp of spirulina in the powder form
- Add one pinch of grounded cinnamon
- Add one pinch of ginger in the form of powder

Directions:

Take a blender and the add ingredients in the blender. Blend these ingredients for a few minutes to get a smooth and creamy texture. Use a scraper to scrape down all sides of blender as per your need.

Recipe No. 8: Ginger-Orange Green Smoothie Recipe

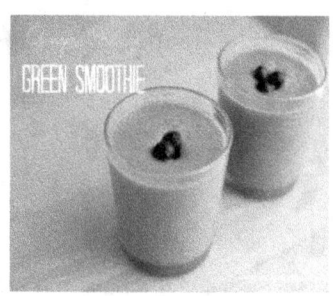

Preparation time: 6 minutes

Servings: 3 glass

Ingredients to add:

- 1 1/2 cups of plan water
- 4 cup of spinach
- 4 romaine leaves if you want
- 2 large oranges
- 2 peeled bananas
- 1 inch of fresh ginger
- 1 peeled cucumber

Directions:

Take a blender and add every ingredient in it. Blend these ingredients to get a smooth and creamy texture.

Recipe No. 9: Green Skin Cleanser

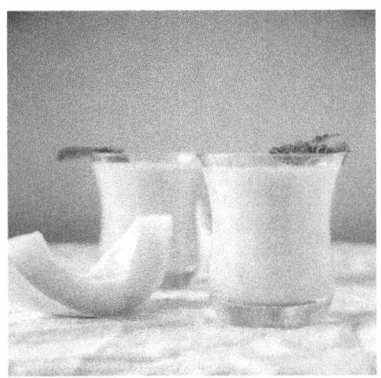

Time required: 9 minutes

Servings: 3 glass of smoothies

Ingredients:

- Spinach: 1 ½ cups
- Coconut water 1 cup
- Frozen Pineapple only 1 cup
- Chopped and corded ¼ slice of Avocado
- Ice cubes: 5 to 7

Directions:

In first step you have to blend coconut milk and spinach to make a smooth paste. Second step follows addition of the remaining ingredients and blend them once again to make a smooth mixture. Enjoy the cooled smoothie.

Recipe No. 10: Tropical Green Smoothie

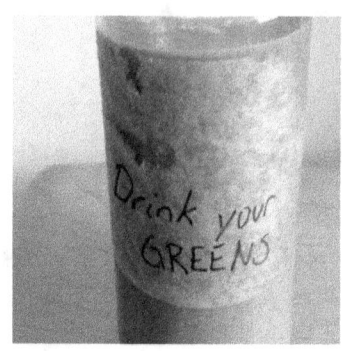

Preparation time: 7 - 9 minutes

Servings: 3 glass of smoothie

Ingredients:

- Pineapple chunks only 2 cups
- Kale 2 cups
- Almond Milk: ¾ cups
- Peeled bananas only 2

Directions:

Take a powerful blender and add all ingredients in this blender. Blend these ingredients for a few minutes at high speed to get a smooth and creamy blend. Use a scraper to scrape down all sides of blender as per your need. If the smoothie is too thick, you can add extra milk. You can store the leftover smoothie in the refrigerator for almost 8 to 10 hours.

Recipe No.11: Blueberry Mint Green Smoothie

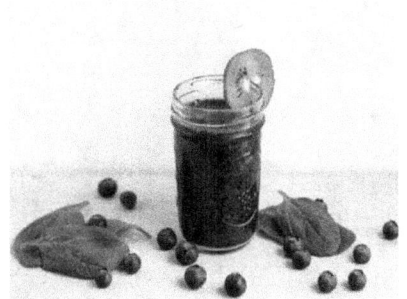

Time for preparation: 6 minutes

Portions: 3 smoothies

Ingredients:

- 3 mint leaves
- 1 glass of coconut water
- 1 cup of ice
- 2 cups of spinach
- 2 cups of blueberry
- Only 1 kiwi

Directions:

Put all ingredients in a blender and mix it up. Make a smooth paste.

Recipe No. 12: Spring Detox Smoothie

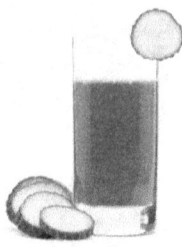

Time for preparation: 5 minutes

Servings: 2 glass of smoothie

Ingredients:

- Pour 1 cup of chilled green tea.
- Add 1 cup of cilantro
- Add 1 cup of kale
- Add 1 cup of cucumber
- Add 1 cup of pineapple
- Squeeze the juice of 1 lemon
- Add 1 tbsp. of grated fresh ginger.
- Add ½ avocado

Directions:

Take a blender and add all the ingredient in the blender. Blend these ingredients to get a smooth and creamy texture.

Chapter 5: Success Stories Of People Benefiting From Smoothie Detox Drinks

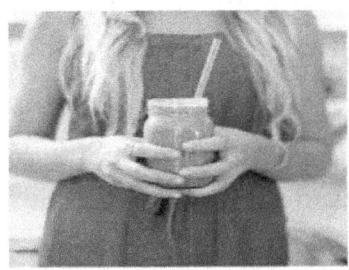

Green smoothie drinks work wonders! From making one active to improving their immune system, from providing nutrients to burning the extra fat. What good they don't do? Let's see what people have to say about them. Here's a few real life success stories:

Brandy's sugar addiction is gone!

Brandy never thought that she would get over her 'sugar addiction' any time sooner in her life but then she had her first detox smoothie in the year 2004. Although at first she did not like the taste but ever since she has discovered the right proportion of the ingredients, she has not been able to part herself from the green delight! Being a sugar person, her diet consisted of all the elements that were enough to make one's belly fat and round. She was worried if she continued in this direction, one day she will become obese and this was her biggest fear. The only way to prevent herself from getting out of shape was to cut off the unnecessary sugar in her diet and there she was introduced to the green smoothies- her only messiah! She noticed that her craving for the sugars was reduced as the green smoothies provided her with the right ingredients that her body needed. She found herself more drawn to the smoothies than to the candies, chocolates and the cakes. She replaced refined sugar with the natural sugar found in fruits and vegetables in her diet and was finally able to cast aside her sugar addiction and the worries she carried on her mind regarding her unhealthy diet. She works as a bartender and makes green smoothies for her customers who seem to like them a lot. She has been inspiring many lives since then and she wishes to continue doing so.

Bonnie says he will never diet again!

How is it like to be an overweight adult? Most of us have some vague idea but Bonnie knew what exactly to say. He weighed 280kg, had been on a weight watch and followed nearly every diet section on all the magazines blindly but anything that he ever tried never seemed to help him. Besides that, he also suffered from high blood pressure, inflammatory disease and joint pain. On top of that, his wrinkles were getting worse day by day which added to his low self-esteem. His diet consisted of all the junk in the world and he would not stop eating on the cheat days of his diet which he had been following fanatically. Because of his weight issues he got divorced and was living a miserable life until he found the green smoothies which according to him are his new lifestyle.

Bonnie has lost 18.2kg after adapting to the new lifestyle he has chosen for himself, in the last 9 months. He is happily remarried again and wishes to reach his ideal weight by continuing the intake. His skin has started to glow and the wrinkles have started to fade away. His joint pain has gone and he barely uses any medication for the pain and the high BP now. He is thankful for the 'fast food' that the nature has provided him with. He is more active, lively and confident than ever. He wishes to reach his ideal weight and is determined to do so.

Dalla has experienced the maximum benefits!

Dalla tried juicing for many years and found it very expensive and time taking as it required costly fruits and the blender cleaning and the juice filtering took forever. At first, he was attracted to the green smoothies because it did not take much of his time in preparation.

When he began taking the green smoothies he weighed 129.3kg. A year later, he weighed 108.9kg. Out of so many benefits, he had experienced a positive change in his bowel movements i.e., he cured the constipation which he had been suffering from for many years, his energy level was increased i.e., now he could work for hours without getting fatigued, he felt satiety after drinking the smoothie and it also served his cravings well in the afternoon, he improved his digestion and on top of all he does not worry about his nutrimental needs anymore as the smoothie provides him with all the nutrients that his body needs. He was also worried about his lean muscles that made him look a little girlish which not only improved as a result of the exercise he had been doing for years but he prefers giving credit to the smoothies as well because the muscle strength only got better after he started using the smoothie. He has been taking them once a day for the past one year. His main aim was to lose the weight and save the time but then he witnessed other benefits as well so he decided to make it a routine. His new goal is not to lose more weight but to increase his overall thin muscle mass. His idea is to start in taking green smoothies twice a day somewhat than just once in the morning. He seems to be satisfied with everything that it does to him. He strongly recommends using smoothie not only with the aim to lose weight but to improve the overall health as well, as it has more benefits than what one can expect.

Chapter 6: Smoothie Recipes

Apples And Cream Smoothie

Ingredients

1 cup of unsweetened apple sauce

1 cup of fat-free or low-fat milk

Ground cinnamon

2 cups of vanilla low-fat ice cream

¼ teaspoon of ground apple pie spice

Directions

[1]pour the low-fat ice cream, apple sauce and apple pie spice into your blender

[2]blend the ingredients until the mixture is smooth

[3]add the milk to the blender and blend further

[4]pour out the smoothie into suitable glass cups and garnish each cup with ground cinnamon

[5]serve

Apple Carrot Quencher

Ingredients

1 banana

½ cup of apple juice

2 cups of carrot juice

6 ounces of frozen yoghurt

Directions

[1]slice up the banana into smaller pieces

[2]pour the slices banana, carrot juice, apple juice and frozen yoghurt into a blender

[3]blend the ingredients until the resulting mixture appears smooth

[4]pour into tall glass cups and serve

Avocado Avalanche

Ingredients

1 cup of ice

2 teaspoons of condensed milk

1 large avocado

Directions

[1]scrape out all the avocado and pour into your blender

[2]add the condensed milk and cup of ice

[3]blend the ingredients until the ice cubes are crushed and the mixture becomes smooth

[4]serve

Avocado Banana Berry Smoothie

Ingredients

½ of a large avocado

Pinch of Allspice

Pinch of Cardamom

1 ½ frozen bananas

5 fresh/frozen strawberries

¾ cup of non-fat soy milk

Directions

[1] scoop out the avocado and pour into the blender

[2] add the allspice, cardamom, frozen bananas, strawberries and soy milk to the blender

[3] blend all ingredients till they attain your desired level of smoothness

[4] serve

Banana Blueberry Smoothie

Ingredients

1 cup of plain yoghurt

2 bananas

½ cup of blueberries

Directions

[1]slice up the bananas and place them in the refrigerator till they become frozen

[2]once the bananas harden, pour them in the blender

[3]slice up the berries and pour them into the blender along with the plain yoghurt

[4]blend the ingredients until they become smooth

[5]serve

Banana Orange Twist

Ingredients

½ cup of water

½ cup of milk

½ of a banana

¼ teaspoon of vanilla

3 ounces of frozen orange juice concentrate

6 ice cubes

Directions

[1]pour the first five ingredients listed above into your blender

[2]blend the ingredients for about 20 seconds

[3]add the ice cubes into the blender and blend for about two minutes

[4]serve

Banana Split Smoothie

Ingredients

5 frozen strawberries

1 cup of non-fat milk

½ cup of pineapple chunks

1 ½ cups of frozen banana slices

2 tablespoons of sweetened cocoa powder

Directions

[1] transfer the non-fat milk into the blender

[2] next, add the cocoa powder followed by the pineapple and frozen banana slices

[3] blend the ingredients till they become smooth

[4] serve

Berry Blue Smoothie

Ingredients

3 tablespoons of honey

2 cups of fresh or frozen blueberries

6 ounces of cups milk

8 ounces of low-fat vanilla yogurt

12 ounces of pineapple juice

16 ice cubes

Directions

[1]pour all of the first five ingredients listed above into your blender

[2]blend until they become smooth

[3]next, add the ice cubes by putting in two cubes at a time while the blender is still running

[4]add two cubes repeatedly until all the ice cubes have been used up

[5]blend further till the mixture becomes smooth

[6]serve

Blackberry Smoothie

Ingredients

1 large banana

½ cup of plain yoghurt

¾ cup of apple juice

1 ½ cups of frozen blackberries

Directions

[1]empty both the yoghurt and apple juice into your blender and stir

[2]slice up the banana into smaller pieces and add them to the blender along with the frozen blackberries

[3]blend until the mixture becomes smooth

[4]serve

Blueberry Maple Smoothie

Ingredients

1 tablespoon of maple syrup

3/4 cups of low-fat milk

1 cup of low-fat blueberry yogurt

½ teaspoon of cinnamon

2 cups of frozen blueberries

Directions

[1]empty the maple syrup, milk, yoghurt and cinnamon into your blender

[2]add the blueberries to the contents of the blender

[3]blend until it turns smooth

[4]serve

Cappuccino Smoothie

Ingredients

Ground Cinnamon

Whipped cream

1 ½ cups of milk

6 cups of ice

2 cups freshly-brewed double strength coffee

1 pint coffee ice cream

Directions

[1]empty all of the coffee, milk, ice cream and ice cubes into your blender

[2]blend the ingredients until they become smooth

[3]pour out the drink into suitable mugs

[4]garnish each serving with whipped cream and top it up with ground cinnamon

[5]serve

Cherry Vanilla Smoothie

Ingredients

2 cups of frozen cherries

1 cup of frozen vanilla yogurt

1 cup of apple juice

Directions

[1]empty the frozen yoghurt and apple juice into a blender and stir

[2]pour in the cherries and blend until they become smooth

[3]serve

Chocolate Banana Smoothie

Ingredients

½ cup of non-fat milk

1 frozen banana

6 ounces of fat-free vanilla or cherry frozen yogurt

2 tablespoons of Hershey's chocolate syrup

Directions

[1] pour all of the ingredients listed above into a blender

[2] blend until it attains your preferred level of smoothness

[3] serve

Double Apple Smoothie

Ingredients

2 bananas, sliced

1 green apple, sliced

1 red apple, sliced

12 frozen strawberries

2 cups of apple juice

Directions

[1]add the 2 bananas to your blender followed by the green apple

[2]next, add the red apple and strawberries

[3]pour in the apple juice and blend all ingredients at high speed until the mixture becomes smooth

[4]serve

Frozen Fruit Smoothie

Ingredients

2 cups of milk

¼ cup of orange juice

2 tablespoons of honey

½ cup of frozen bananas

½ cup of frozen peaches

½ cup of frozen strawberries

Directions

[1]add all of the above ingredients into a blender

[2]mix the ingredients at high speed till it becomes smooth

[3]serve

Fruit Salad Smoothie

Ingredients

2 cups of skimmed evaporated milk(chilled)

½ of a banana

1 teaspoon of vanilla

1 medium ripe peach

¾ cup of fresh/frozen strawberries

4 teaspoons of frozen orange juice concentrate

6 ice cubes

Ground Cinnamon

Directions

[1]add all of the above ingredients into a blender

[2]mix the ingredients at high speed till it becomes smooth

[3]with the blender still running, add the ice cubes, one at a time, to the blender

[4]blend further until it's smooth

[5]pour out into glass cups and garnish each serving with ground cinnamon

[6]serve

Guava Smoothie

Ingredients

1 cup of peach sorbet

1 frozen banana

1 cup of frozen strawberries

1 can of guava nectar

Directions

[1] empty all of the ingredients into a blender

[2] mix at high speed till it becomes smooth

[3] serve

Hawaiian Silk Smoothie

Ingredients

1 tablespoon of maple syrup

2 tablespoons of non-fat dry milk

1 cup of soy milk

½ cup of pineapple juice

1 frozen banana

1 tablespoon of coconut milk

Ice cubes

Directions

[1] empty all of the ingredients into a blender

[2] mix at high speed till it becomes smooth

[3] serve

Honey Raspberry Smoothie

Ingredients

1 cup of plain low fat yogurt

2 tablespoons of honey

1 banana

1 cup of frozen raspberries

1 cup of cold skim milk

¼ teaspoon of vanilla

8 ice cubes

Directions

[1]pour half a cup of milk in the blender and add the frozen raspberries

[2]blend at high speed for few minutes till mixture becomes smooth

[3]next, add the yoghurt, honey, banana, vanilla and the remaining half cup of milk into the blender

[4]blend further till it attains smoothness

[5]pour the ice cubes into the blender and blend until ice cubes become crushed and the drink is smooth

[6]serve

Kiwi Cooler

Ingredients

2 cups of pineapple juice

1 cup of sparkling water

5 kiwi fruits

4 large strawberries

4 ice cubes

Directions

[1]first, peel all the kiwis and slice them up into smaller sizes

[2]place the sliced kiwis in the blender and pour in the pineapple juice and ice cubes

[3]blend ingredients till it becomes smooth

[4]add the cup of sparkling water and stir

[5]serve and garnish with strawberries

Lemon Lime Smoothie

Ingredients

1 scoop of lemon sherbet

1 scoop of lime sherbet

Half a banana

10 ounces of lemon lime soda

2 ounces of lemons

2 ounces of lime

2/3 cup of granulated sugar

1 cup of ice

Directions

[1] empty all of the ingredients into a blender

[2]mix at high speed till it becomes smooth

[3]serve

Lemonade Sweet Tart Smoothie

Ingredients

1 cup of milk

1 cup of water

6 ounces of frozen lemonade concentrate

¼ cup of sugar

1 teaspoon of vanilla extract

10 ice cubes

Directions

[1] empty all of the ingredients into a blender

[2]mix at high speed till it becomes smooth

[3]serve

Mango Smoothie

Ingredients

¼ cup of non-fat vanilla yogurt

¾ teaspoon of vanilla extract

Pinch of salt

Fresh mint sprigs

1 ripe mango, peeled, chopped

¾ cup of skim milk, chilled

3-4 ice cubes

Directions

[1] peel the mango and scrape it into the blender with the chilled milk, yogurt, vanilla extract, salt and ice cubes

[2] blend until the mixture is smooth

[3] serve and garnish with mint sprigs

Mexican Smoothie

Ingredients

¼ teaspoon of cayenne

¼ cup of chopped onions

1 cup of tomato juice

½ teaspoon of chopped jalapeno pepper

½ cup of chopped parsley

2 cloves of garlic, peeled

Directions

[1] empty all of the ingredients into a blender

[2] mix at high speed till it becomes smooth

[3] serve

Orange Pineapple Smoothie

Ingredients

Half of a banana

¼ teaspoon of ginger root (peeled, grated)

½ cup of orange juice

½ cup of pineapple juice

2 ice cubes

Directions

[1] empty all of the ingredients into a blender

[2]mix at high speed till it becomes smooth

[3]serve

Organic Smoothie

Ingredients

1 banana

2 cups of organic orange juice

1 cup of frozen organic strawberries

½ cup of frozen organic blueberries

Directions

[1] empty all of the ingredients into a blender

[2]mix at high speed till it becomes smooth

[3]serve

Papaya Smoothie

Ingredients

2 ripe papayas

½ cup of vanilla frozen yogurt

½ cup of orange juice

Directions

[1]first, peel the papaya and remove the seeds

[2]chop up the papaya into smaller sizes and pour into the blender

[3]add yogurt and orange juice

[4]blend until the mixture is smooth

[5]serve

Peaches And Dreams Smoothie

Ingredients

4 large strawberries

1 banana

10 ounces of apple cider

1/8 teaspoons of cinnamon

4 slices of peach

Directions

[1] pour all of the ingredients into a blender

[2]mix at high speed till it becomes smooth

[3]serve

Peanut Butter Smoothie

Ingredients

1 cup of vanilla ice cream

¼ cup of peanut butter

1 cup of milk

Directions

[1] pour all of the ingredients into a blender

[2] mix at high speed till it becomes smooth enough

[3] serve

Peanut Butter Sundae Smoothie

Ingredients

1/3 cup of milk

¼ teaspoon of wheat germ

¼ cup of smooth peanut butter

2 tablespoons of honey

3 cups of vanilla ice milk

Directions

[1]combine the milk, honey and peanut butter together in a saucepan

[2]stir and apply low heat to the saucepan while stirring the ingredients frequently

[3]once the peanut butter has dissolved, remove the saucepan from the heat source and add the wheat germ and ice milk

[4]stir and

[5]serve chilled

Peppermint Smoothie

Ingredients

1 teaspoon of vanilla extract

4 scoops of peppermint ice cream

1 ½ cups of milk

2 drops of peppermint extract

Directions

[1] pour all of the ingredients into a blender

[2]mix at high speed till it becomes smooth

[3]serve

Pina Banana Smoothie

Ingredients

½ cup of pineapple chunks

1 ½ cups of frozen banana slices

1 cup of pineapple juice

1/3 cup of coconut milk

Directions

[1]combine both the pineapple juice and coconut milk together in the blender and stir

[2]next, add the banana slices and pineapple to the blender

[3]blend the ingredients until they become smooth

[4]serve

Pina Colada Smoothie

Ingredients

2 teaspoons of shredded coconut

¼ cup of fresh chopped pineapples

1 frozen banana

1 cup of milk or soymilk

Directions

[1] pour all of the ingredients into a blender

[2]mix at high speed till it becomes smooth

[3]serve

Pineapple Papaya Smoothie

Ingredients

1 cup of pineapple chunks

1 ½ cups of frozen papaya chunks

1 cup of orange juice

1 tablespoon of unsweetened shredded coconut

Directions

[1]pour the orange juice in the blender first

[2]add shredded coconut followed by the papaya and pineapple

[3]blend the ingredients until they're smooth

[4]serve

Pink Smoothie Deluxe

Ingredients

1 cup of red grapefruit juice

1 cup of orange juice

2 cups of sliced bananas

1 ½ cups of frozen strawberries

1 cup of ice cubes

Directions

[1] pour all of the ingredients into a blender

[2]mix at high speed till it becomes smooth

[3]serve

Purple Passion Smoothie

Ingredients

1/3 cup of blueberries

1/3 cup of strawberries

1 banana

1 cup of non-fat yogurt

2/3 cup of ice

Directions

[1] pour all of the ingredients into a blender

[2] mix until it becomes smooth

[3] serve

Rainbow Smoothie

Ingredients

Half of a banana

4 ounces of strawberries

½ cup of ice

10 ounces of apple-cranberry juice

2 ounces of pineapple chunks

2 scoops of rainbow sherbet

Directions

[1] pour all of the ingredients into a blender

[2] mix until it becomes smooth

[3] serve

Raspberry Orange Smoothie

Ingredients

2 cups of fresh raspberries

1 cup of frozen orange juice concentrate

1 cup of ice cubes

2 cups of milk

2 cups of plain yogurt

1 teaspoon of vanilla extract

Directions

[1] pour all of the ingredients into a blender

[2] mix until it becomes smooth

[3] serve

Raspberry Watermelon Smoothie

Ingredients

½ pint of raspberries

2 cups of seeded watermelon chunks

1 tablespoon of Sugar

1 cup of ice cubes

Directions

[1] pour all of the ingredients into a blender

[2]mix until it becomes smooth

[3]serve

Smoothie Power Shake

Ingredients

½ cup of cantaloupe

1 tablespoon of peanut butter

1 cup of non-fat soy milk

½ cup of orange juice

1 banana

½ cup of strawberries, (fresh or frozen)

Directions

[1] pour all of the ingredients into a blender

[2] mix until it becomes smooth

[3] serve

Strawberry Banana Smoothie

Ingredients

4 strawberries

1 banana

½ cup of skim milk

½ cup of apple juice

Directions

[1] pour all of the ingredients into a blender

[2] mix until it becomes smooth

[3] serve

Strawberry Blueberry Smoothie

Ingredients

1 frozen banana (peeled)

1 ½ cup of milk

½ cup of frozen blueberries

1 cup of frozen strawberries

½ cup of frozen vanilla or strawberry yogurt

Directions

[1] pour all of the ingredients into a blender

[2]mix until it becomes smooth

[3]serve

Strawberry Kiwi Smoothie

Ingredients

½ cup of frozen strawberries

1 cup of frozen banana slices

3 peeled kiwi fruits

¾ cup of pineapple juice

Directions

[1] pour all of the ingredients into a blender

[2] mix until it becomes smooth

[3] serve

Strawberry Lemonade Smoothie

Ingredients

¼ cup of sugar

¼ cup of cold water

½ cup of freshly squeezed lemon juice

3 cups of frozen strawberries (sliced)

2 cups of ice

Directions

[1]first combine the water and lemon juice in the blender

[2]add sugar, strawberries and ice

[3]blend ingredients till they appear smooth

[4]serve

Strawberry Raspberry Smoothie

Ingredients

1 cup of frozen strawberries

1 cup of frozen raspberries

1 banana

1 ½ cups of orange juice

Directions

[1]empty the orange juice into a blender

[2]add all the other ingredients and blend for a few minutes until the mixture comes out smooth

[3]serve

Strawberry Sunrise Smoothie

Ingredients

¼ cup of apple juice

8 ounces of vanilla yogurt

½ cup of frozen strawberries

1 frozen banana (chopped)

Directions

[1]empty the apple juice into a blender

[2]add all the other ingredients and blend for a few minutes until the mixture comes out smooth

[3]serve

Tangerine Dreams Smoothie

Ingredients

2 ripe bananas

1 cup of tangerine juice

1 ripe papaya, seeded, peeled and sliced

Directions

[1] pour all of the ingredients into a blender

[2]mix until it becomes smooth

[3]serve

Tropical Fling Smoothie

Ingredients

½ cup of ripe pineapple (peeled and cut up)

½ cup of mango (peeled and cut up)

½ cup of milk

½ cup of plain yogurt

2 teaspoons of fresh lime juice

Ground sugar

Directions

[1] pour all of the ingredients into a blender

[2]mix until it becomes smooth

[3]add ground sugar to sweeten if desired

[4]serve

Wacky Watermelon Smoothie

Ingredients

½ cup of plain yogurt

1 tablespoon of sugar

½ teaspoon of ground ginger

2 cups of watermelon (seeded and cut up)

1/8 teaspoon of almond extract

1 cup of ice

Directions

[1] pour all of the ingredients into a blender

[2]mix until it becomes smooth

[3]serve

Zippy Pineapple Carrot Smoothie

Ingredients

1 carrot, peeled and sliced

1/3 cup of pineapple juice

1inchpiece of ginger, peeled and minced

½ cup of pineapple chunks

1 cup of soy milk, any flavor

Honey

Directions

[1] pour all of the ingredients into a blender

[2]mix until it becomes smooth

[3]serve

Conclusion

Now a days, losing weight is one of the biggest challenge. For some people, not following a right diet plan is the reason while for others the diet itself surrenders after an opportunity to eat. The nutritionist have found an ultimate solution for this problem and it is called 'green smoothie' which is a blend of raw fruits and vegetables that provides you with all the right nutrients that your body needs; minerals, vitamins, fibers and water all in one cup of a green mixture. It not only helps one to lose weight but it also comes with several other health benefits as well such as improved immune system, glowing skin and improved muscle mass. It is easy on the pocket and it hardly takes 10 minutes to prepare. For children, who do not like to eat veggies, green smoothies are the best way to make them develop the taste, besides that it fulfills the nutrients requirement of the body. One may use it as part of regular meal or may also use it as a diet plan. If you want to lose more weight in less time then you have grabbed the right book. Follow the easy-to-make recipes and get ready to feel light, active and healthy again. For better results, replace the soft drinks with natural green smoothies, take it twice a day, use fruits to improve the taste and consult your dietician for more guidance. Remember not to ever compromise on health. It cannot be bought!

Part 2

Introduction

This book contains proven steps and strategies on how to include the amazing green smoothies in your diet. Aren't you a smoothie lover? Are you worried about your increasing weight? Are you tired of the junk food? Do you want to make revolutionary changes in your lifestyle? If the answers of these questions are yes, then what are you waiting for? Grab this book and open new doors of freshness, fitness and health. This book contains a detailed discussion on the benefits and effects of the green smoothies on our health and lifestyle. You will be amazed to know that how these simple green smoothies can make great improvements in your health. You will be pleased after having this book. This book is really going to change your perception about the green smoothies. This book contains proven steps and strategies on how to include The amazing green smoothies in your diet. It also includes 25 amazing green smoothie recipes which are quick and easy to make. The recipes are simple and are one of their kind.

Thanks again for downloading this book, I hope you enjoy it!

Green Smoothies; Drinking
 Your Nutrition A Delicious Way

You must have always enjoyed smoothies, but did you ever consider adding greens and other veggies to it? Undoubtedly, at first it doesn't sound very appealing. However, from the very first day when you will start adding kale, baby spinach, mint and other greens to your usual banana, strawberry and other fruity smoothies, I bet you will be utterly hooked to them. Green smoothie will give you a blast of heavenly taste with a lot of visible positive side effects. On top of that, the green smoothie will help you overcome your cravings for the sweets which in return will aid you to eat less calories and lose weight.

What is Green Smoothie?

Green smoothies, like most of the smoothies, are the beverages that are shaken to combine fruits with the leafy greens such as mustard, spinach, chard, beet greens, bok Choy and other edible leafy greens. You can also add some common vegetables that are not necessarily green such as broccoli, mushrooms or even the carrots. The idea of adding raw greens to your usual yummy tasting smoothies may seem to be a little weird, but once you try, it will leave you with barely tasting some greens inside.

Why Bother?

If blast of energy, clear skin and weight loss is something you are after with least efforts involved, adding dark greens to your diet would be the best choice. But like most of the people, it's almost near to impossible to have the greens every day in your meals. To achieve a healthy weight loss putting less effort, it's a great idea to have the greens blended smoothly with your favorite fruits and gulp the whole glass full of healthy nutrients we usually lack in our daily diet. So if you are not much into cooking and not able to get a lot of time spent in the kitchen, a green smoothie is a blessing for you. Keep reading and you will soon realize, how?

Without Even Trying, Have More Greens

The question is how much parsley do you consume in one meal? You may love parsley, but I am sure you just get it sprinkled over your food and that's all for the day. However, in case of a smoothie, things are different. One enchanting handful of parsley would be the amount you are going to consume in a single smoothie even without having the greens overpowered. You won't even realize you just had any green in your usual fruit smoothie.

Get Going!

Health Benefits

Now, when you seem to be a little interested in the concept of this new addition to your life, let's discuss the countless health benefits you are going to have with just a glass of smoothie each day.

An Excellent Way to Increase Raw Green Vegetable Intake

On top of the list, a green smoothie is the best way to consume raw green vegetables that otherwise you are unable to, in a single sitting. For example, you may like sautéed kale or baby spinach and usually have them in your salads, but to extract the maximum nutrition out of these vegetables you need to have them raw. Having a handful of raw spinach or kale seems to be a little weird. So, dump the gorgeous handful of the raw spinach into the blender along with your favorite fruit like banana or the strawberry, add water and just blend until smooth. This is all you have to do every day in this healthy lifestyle.

The normal veg-fruit ratio is 40% vegetable and 60% fruit. However, it is suggested to get started with a little less vegetable and a little more fruit just to get used to the green smoothie. Once you develop the taste you can keep increasing the vegetable ratio.

Easy to Digest

Blending the raw vegetables until smooth you get essentially pre-digested food. This way you feed the body with something that's easily digested and eliminated. The broken down cells of raw vegetables and fruits assimilate the nutrients very quickly into the body. Enzymes in the raw fruits and vegetables help digesting our food. Green smoothie also helps to reduce the inflammation in our body.

Healthy Weight loss

Green smoothies are the power house of certain healthy nutrients that help curb your cravings. You feel full quickly and no more crave for fattening foods. You snack less often than before and the artificial or fattening food intake decreases. The good news is, consequently you will be able to fit into your old jeans you never imagined to button again.

Boost in Energy

When fruits and vegetables are blended together, the nutrients inside them become more absorbable. This makes you feel a lot more alive with a blast of energy. This is how, exercising regularly will become a piece of cake if you drink a glass of green smoothie before getting started with your daily exercise. This is another plus if you want to lose weight.

Stronger Immune System

The high chlorophyll content present in vegetables results in a stronger immune system. Thus, your body strengthens to fight the diseases off. High acidic PH levels of our body lead to diseases and illnesses. Green smoothies also help alkalize our body's blood PH. By neutralizing the acidic environment green smoothies keep you from illness and diseases. Their capability of being high antioxidants the green smoothies prevent from certain types of cancers. People who stay on regular use of green smoothies claim to get sick less often.

Clear Skin and Healthy Hair

Green smoothies do not only benefit your inner body system, but they also make your skin clear and spotless. The blend of fruits and vegetables detoxifies your body and using them for a period of time will make you get rid of your body toxins, eliminating bloating and constipation. You will experience glowing and radiant skin as well as faster hair growth. You will feel no more need to spend lots of money on the cosmetics because the regular intake of green smoothies will grant you with the natural beauty.

A Quick Snack

A glass of rich green smoothie appears to be a very quick snack that you can have anytime you crave for sweets or wanting a quick snack. Needless to say that they are a lot better than your junk food choices like pizzas, sandwiches or other fattening artificial foods. Regular use of green smoothies will keep your body clean from toxins and regulate the bowel movements. You can have them as a snack or even as a breakfast. Being packed with healthy and energizing nutrients you will feel enough energy to sustain your daily functions.

Eliminating waste and adding healthy components to your diet in a smart way will eventually lead you to a healthy life.

Green Smoothies Are Better Than Fresh Juices

It is a common perception that the fresh juices and smoothies are same. In other words, green juices have equal benefits as green smoothies which is totally wrong. Smoothies are made by blending all the ingredients together in a blender. This process keeps all the nutrients of the fruits and vegetables within the drink while juices are extracted from the ingredients through special juice machines. It is a process that extracts the liquid from the fruits or vegetables discarding the rest of the remains. This technique wastes many of the useful components of the fruits and veggies.

Green Smoothies are an Instant Meal

In the green smoothies, all the fruits and vegetables are blended together. This blending makes the digestion very easy and quick. These smoothies are just to be absorbed by the digestive system. This gives the human body an instant and sudden boost in energy unlike the other meals which take 6 hours for the complete digestion of the food. That is why these green smoothies are often called instant meals. The calorie content of these smoothies is equivalent to that of a proper meal, but with less side effects. They contain very little or no amount of fat, which help to burn some extra fat stored in your body without decreasing your energy level.

Green Smoothies Contain the Whole Nutritional Benefits

The difference between the techniques of making smoothies and juices is explained above. People say that the green juices and the juices of other vegetables also have the same effectiveness as the green smoothies have. Green smoothies contain pulp of the fruits or vegetables added. This pulp contains fiber, which increases the ability of this smoothie to get absorbed in the blood. The juices contain a large amount of the sugar present in the fruit or the vegetable. This makes them a pure sweetener and a great concern for the diabetic patients. On the other hand, the fiber in the green smoothies slows down the sugar absorption in the blood. This gives freedom for all the persons who are concerned about their sugar level.

Green Smoothies Can Replace Meals

As it is discussed that the green smoothies contain the whole fruits and vegetables, they are heavy enough to fulfil your hunger in a healthy way. You can replace your breakfast or even lunch with a green smoothie of your choice. All you have to do is to have a green smoothie which is balanced in every way. It should be containing enough calories to keep you going until the next meal, it should have protein and it should be having vegetables which contain antioxidants. You can add calories equivalent to a meal by adding fruits in your green smoothie which contain higher amount of calories like mangoes, banana or grapes. The thick and creamy texture of these smoothies makes you feel like having a proper meal. This is simply a perfect, time saving and satisfying meal for your whole life.

Green Smoothies are Enough to Fulfil Your Hunger and Cravings

Green smoothies contain whole fruits and whole vegetables. The quantity of fruits or vegetables, these smoothies contain are more than you consume during a normal meal. For example, you can add lettuce in your meal as toppings. In this way you just include few leaves while in smoothies you can add any vegetable of your choice in a large quantity comparatively. Moreover, vegetables like kale are added into salads or meals after sautéing or frying. This processing of the vegetables wastes many necessary and important components. On the other hand, the green smoothies contain fresh and raw ingredients to ensure maximum benefits. This makes these smoothies so much important special.

Green Smoothies are Slowly Oxidized as Compared to Green Juices

The green juices contain just the nutrients and extract of the fruits or the vegetables. These nutrients are exposed to oxidation and bacteria which are responsible for fermentation and decaying process. While the green smoothies contain the pulp of the fruits and vegetables. This pulp and fiber protect the nutrients from the oxidation and bacterial attack. This also slows down the oxidation process and the green smoothies last longer. These smoothies can be placed in the refrigerator for two to three days without adding any preservative.

The Ingredients Are Easy to Manage

The green smoothies are composed of fresh and whole fruits and vegetables. The procedure of these green smoothies makes these ingredients easy to manage and clean up after you had your smoothie. You just need to wash and add your favorite ingredients in a blender and blend them together. They have another plus point that there is no waste of these smoothies like you extract the liquids out of the ingredients in green juices and dump the rest of it.

Green Smoothies are Good Antioxidants

Green smoothies can contain many green vegetables such as kale, spinach, cucumber and many others.

These vegetables are rich in antioxidants. Antioxidants are minerals and vitamins and other nutrients which help to repair the damaged cells of the different parts or organs of the human body. These nutrients also slow down the oxidation process. These antioxidants also help the body to get rid of the harmful nutrients which are somehow absorbed in the body during the digestion process. They also help in cleansing of the blood and hence helping the kidneys and liver.

Green Smoothies Are Anti-Aging

From the beginning of time, people always tried different ways to stop aging or to live longer. Many people tried different crazy things and some of them spent their whole lives for this. Well, these were the stories when there were no green smoothies. We will now discuss how the green smoothies are anti-aging and how they help you to live longer.

Aging Effects are Related to the Food We Eat

It is now a known fact that the aging effects are related to the food we eat. This is also a fact that we cannot do anything about our chronological age, but we certainly can do something about our biological age. The more we consume the meaty, spicy foods and the food which is based on animals the more you face the aging effects. Adopting and sticking to the diet which is based on fresh and raw food like vegetables and fruits can help us a lot regarding this. The antioxidants in these types of foods help cleansing the blood and many internal organs. These organs have to do less amount of work and thus increasing their biological life time.

Green Smoothies Help Fight Free Radicals

They say that the aging is directly related to the free radicals. These free radicals are some effects produced in the body when we are exposed to some harmful effects of smoking, pollution, fat containing meats and some other hazardous materials or phenomena. These free radicals effect and damage the healthy cells of our body. The human body naturally has an immune system which fights these free radicals and the effects caused by them. But we feel the heat of this fight when the free radicals are more than the strength of our immune system. In those cases, the food we consume plays a key role. Fresh and raw foods, like these green smoothies are very much effective to boost up our immune system and to fight against the toxic chemicals that somehow enter our body.

Biological Aging is Related to New and Healthy Cell Generation

The aging can be slowed down or in other words the effects of aging can be prevented if your body regularly replaces the dead and damaged cells of the different organs and parts of your body. This only happens if your body has a stronger and effective immune system. The immune system fights the diseases which attack the body and helps repair the damages. The green smoothies contain nutrients which are necessary for a stronger immune system. These easy to make and digest smoothies provides an instant and quick boost to the immune system. The effects of these smoothies can be observed and seen within one or two days of including them to your diet.

Some Daily Life Benefits Of Green Smoothies

The food we eat with spices and various cooking methods has many harmful effects. It contains many processed ingredients. These processed foods are somehow the cause of diseases like cancer and heart diseases. These diseases can be prevented by adopting a diet which is based on unprocessed foods. These unprocessed foods are many fruits and vegetables. You have to make these fruits and vegetables a regular part of your diet. Adding 2, 3 raw fruits and vegetables in your diet will be amazed and you will opt for more. The best way to include these amazing vegetables and fruits in your diet is to blend them together and consume as a raw smoothie or green smoothie. No cooking or processing is required you just have to blend the ingredients together and enjoy.

The Same Quantity of This Smoothie Gives More Energy Comparatively

Your diet contains all types of eatables and food materials. Every eatable has its own time which is required for its digestion. In this way the food is not properly digested because some food is digested early and some is digested later. Due to this the human body is unable to obtain all of the energy that is available in the food. In scientific language we can say that the food is not much efficient. This is mainly due to the processed food present in our diet. These processed foods give you a short boost in energy and leave you lazy and with low energy level after that. On the other hand, the green smoothies contain the raw fruits and vegetables. These fruits and vegetables and all of the other ingredients are not processed and cooked. Cooking these vegetables can destroy various important and healthy nutrients. Because of the rawness of the ingredients, it is easier for the digestive system to digest them and obtain maximum benefits out of it. These green smoothies have a huge advantage over the other foods in this regard.

You Need to Get Rid of the Toxins Accumulating Inside Your Body

Along with the healthy nutrients, our body absorbs some other nutrients which are stored inside the body. With the passage of time, these nutrients turn themselves into toxic materials. The human body naturally has a proper system to get rid of these harmful materials. These materials are thrown out of the body, but sometimes, when these toxic materials are large in quantity, the human body fails to get rid of them. These green smoothies contain vegetables, which are rich in antioxidants. These antioxidants are absorbed by the blood and then they remove those toxic materials from the body. These smoothies also help to strengthen the immune system which prevents the attack of diseases in the body. The effect of these fantastic green smoothies can also be seen from the skin. The skin starts looking fresh and glowing when these smoothies are a regular part of your daily lifestyle.

Your Cravings for Fast Foods and Processed Food Will Be Reduced

The longer you expose your body to these natural and beneficial foods like green smoothies, the more you start liking them. The positive effects of these smoothies can be seen from the day first. With so many benefits, you will never carve for the processed and fast foods. You will feel like doing a sin while having these fast and processed foods after knowing all the harmful effects of them. You will always go for these green smoothies for your snacks, desserts and other cravings. You will never feel yourself hungry for chocolates and snacks and these green smoothies will never let you down.

You Will Never Need to Force Your Children to Eat Vegetables

Children of all of the ages, love smoothies. This is a great way to introduce your children to the vegetables. Now you don't need to force your children to eat the vegetables. You just need to add the healthy vegetables in a blender with some delicious fruits and blend them together to create some happiness. Simply increase the ratio of the fruits in these green smoothies and they will love them without knowing that these are made from green vegetables.

Green Smoothies Can Be Taken Before or After Exercise and Workout

The health and nutritional benefits of green smoothies are fact, now after all of this discussion. A cup of green smoothies is a cup of nutrients and happiness. This is a source of instant energy which helps you to do some workout. These smoothies are helpful before or after doing an exercise to get or regain the lost energy in the process. The green smoothies leave a refreshing effect on your mind and body. The instant strength can be felt in your muscles right after a little time after consuming them.

There is a Lot of Room for Varieties

There is a lot of room for variation in these green smoothies. You can use different fruits like strawberries, blueberries, banana, mango and many more. These fruits are responsible for the deliciousness and tastiness in the smoothies. The other part, the vegetables can also be varied with the mood and requirement. Kale, spinach and cucumber are the famous vegetables that are used in green smoothies. These vegetables are responsible for all of the health benefits of green smoothies. In this way, these green smoothies are a complete, trustable and reliable diet.

Green Smoothies are Helpful to Burn Fat

The whole fruits and vegetables in the green smoothies are heavy enough to satisfy your hunger. These fruits and vegetables are rich in nutrients, but are free of the saturated fats. The saturated fats are the fats, which are stored by the body under our skin. By excluding the fats in the diet, our body will refer to the stored fat for its needs. This allows losing some of the stored fat, which was responsible for the obesity. You will find yourself fit and light but you need to be determined and stick to these green smoothies. Green smoothies are the names of a habit, once you start having them, you will never be able to leave them for your whole life. They will become a kind of an addiction, a healthy and beneficial one.

Recipes Of Green Smoothies

This chapter of the book contains the recipes of the green smoothies. All of the recipes are in simple words to make them able to be understood easily. These recipes can be made in no time and with very little effort. One might wonder that how these easy and simple drinks can be of so many benefits. The impact of these smoothies will be huge on your life. These smoothies can change your whole lifestyle. You will be wanting more after observing the amazing effects of these smoothies on your health. Just follow the easy instructions and enjoy!

Coconut & Watermelon Smoothie

Ingredients:

2 cups watermelon, cubed

1 cucumber, sliced

2 tablespoons honey

1 handful mint leaves

2 cups coconut water

2 lemons (peeled)

A pinch of ginger powder

Directions:

- In a blender, add all ingredients and blend till smooth and frothy.
- Pour into 2 glasses and serve.

Avocado Smoothie

Ingredients:

1 avocado, sliced

½ cup frozen raspberries

¾ cup orange juice

¾ cup raspberry juice

Directions:

- In a blender, add all ingredients and blend till smooth and frothy.
- Pour into a glass and serve.

Cabbage With Berry Smoothie

Ingredients:

¼ red cabbage

½ cup fresh raspberries

½ cup fresh blueberries

1 cucumber, sliced

2 cups fresh red apple juice

A pinch of cinnamon

Directions:

- In a blender, add cabbage, cucumber, raspberries, blueberries and apple juice and blend till smooth.
- Sprinkle with cinnamon.
- Serve.

Green Leaf Smoothie

Ingredients:
3 kale leaves
½ cup spinach leaves
1 cucumber, sliced
1 fennel head
2 cups water
1 slices ginger root
2 tablespoons lemon juice

Directions:
- In a blender, add kale, spinach, cucumber, fennel, water, ginger and lemon juice and blend till smooth.
- Serve.

Simple Green Protein Smoothie

Ingredients:

1½ cups pineapple chunks

½ bananas

½ cup Greek yogurt

2 kale leaves

2 cups baby spinach

1 cup water

1 teaspoon honey

Directions:

- In a blender, add all ingredients and blend till smooth and frothy.
- Pour into a glass and serve.

Vanilla Yogurt Smoothie

Ingredients:

6 ounces vanilla yogurt

1/2 cup green grapes, seedless

1 cup spinach

1 cup soy milk

1 cup blueberries

1 tablespoon flaxseed oil

Directions:

- In a blender, add all ingredients and blend till smooth and frothy.

- Pour into a glass and serve.

Carrot Smoothie

Ingredients:

1 ½ cup carrot, chopped

½ cup pear, chopped

1/2 cup baby spinach

2 cups apple juice

1 teaspoon ginger powder

Directions:

- In a blender, add all ingredients and blend till smooth and frothy.
- Pour into 2 glasses and serve.

Grapefruit Smoothie

Ingredients:

2 cups fresh grapefruit juice

1 banana

1 cup baby spinach

1 tablespoon honey

Directions:

- In a blender, add all ingredients and blend till smooth.
- Pour into a glass and serve.

Papaya Smoothie

Ingredients:

¼ cup papaya, chopped

4 celery stalks

¼ cup green cabbage, chopped

1 carrot, chopped

1 cup coconut water

Directions:

- In a blender, add all ingredients and blend till smooth and frothy.
- Pour into a glass and serve.

Almond Smoothie

Ingredients:
½ cup almond milk
1/4 cup spinach
2 tablespoons avocado, sliced
1 tablespoon mint leaves
1 tablespoon flaxseed
¼ cup strawberries

Directions:
- In a blender, add all ingredients and blend till smooth and frothy.
- Pour into a glass and serve.

Celery & Tomato Smoothie

Ingredients:

2 celery stalks

2 fresh tomatoes, sliced

1 cup coconut water

4 ice cubes

Salt and pepper

Directions:

- In a blender, add all ingredients and blend till smooth.
- Pour into a glass and serve.

Beet Green Smoothie

Ingredients:

2 cups beet greens, chopped

1 large apple, sliced

1 banana, sliced

2 cups water

Directions:

- In a blender, add all ingredients and blend till smooth.
- Pour into 2 glasses and serve.

Zucchini Smoothie

Ingredients:

½ cup organic zucchini, chopped

½ cup parsley leaves

2 stalks celery

½ cup pineapple

2 cups pineapple juice

Directions:

- In a blender, add all ingredients and blend till smooth.
- Pour into 2 glasses and serve.

Green Aloe Juice

Ingredients:

1 large fennel bulb

2 large oranges

2 cucumber slices

1fl ounce Aloe juice

6 ice cubes

Directions:

- In a blender, add all ingredients and blend till smooth.
- Pour into a glass and serve.

Anti Aging Smoothie

Ingredients:

3 cups coconut water

¼ cup strawberries

1/2 cup coconut milk

2 tablespoons chia seeds

2 cups baby spinach

1 cucumber, sliced

1 scoop of greens powder

1 teaspoon honey

Ice cubes

Directions:
- In a blender, add all ingredients and blend till smooth and frothy.
- Pour into 2 glasses and serve.

Green Smoothie

Ingredients:

1 cup organic frozen blueberries

3 stalks of kale

1 honey crisp apple

1 banana

½ cup water

1 teaspoon lemon juice

Ice cubed

Directions:

- In a blender, add all ingredients and blend till smooth and frothy.
- Pour into 2 glasses and serve.

Dr. Oz's Green Smoothie

Ingredients:

3 carrots, sliced

2 apples, sliced

1 orange juice

1 lime juice

2 cups spinach

¼ cup cucumber, sliced

¼ cup celery

¼ cup parsley

¼ cup mint

1 tablespoon lemon

1cup pineapple juice

Directions:
- In a blender, add all ingredients and blend till smooth and frothy.
- Pour into3 glasses and serve.

Healthy Skin Smoothie

Ingredients:

5 stalks of celery

1 apple, peeled

2 tablespoons spinach

½ a cucumber, sliced

1 cup water

Directions:

- In a blender, add all ingredients and blend till smooth and frothy.
- Pour into a glass and serve.

Antioxidant Smoothie

Ingredients:

1 cup blueberries

¼ cup water

1 cup spinach

¼ cup cucumber, sliced

½ banana

¼ cup pomegranate juice

1 cup ice cubed

Directions:
- In a blender, add all ingredients and blend till smooth and frothy.
- Pour into a glass and serve.

Berry Medley Smoothie

Ingredients:

1 cup organic spinach

¾ cup frozen berries

¼ avocado

1 teaspoon unsweetened coconut flakes

1 teaspoon chia seeds

8 ounces almond milk

1 teaspoon ground flax meal

Directions:

- In a blender, add all ingredients and blend till smooth and frothy.
- Pour into a glass and serve.

Vitamin C Smoothie

Ingredients:

2 fresh oranges, juiced

1 tomato

1 cucumber, sliced

1 cup strawberries

1/2 cantaloupe

Directions:

- In a blender, add all ingredients and blend till smooth.
- Pour into 2 glasses and serve.

Healthy Hair Smoothie

Ingredients:

1 cup coconut water

2 cups spinach

1 handful walnuts

1 cup blueberries

1 tablespoon raw cacao

1 teaspoon coconut oil

Directions:

- In a blender, add all ingredients and blend till smooth and frothy.
- Pour into a glass and serve.

Super Detox Green Smoothie

Ingredients:

2 celery stalks, chopped

1 apple, seeded, chopped

1 cucumber, chopped

2 kale leaves, chopped

2 tablespoons spinach

1 tablespoon parsley, chopped

1 tablespoon cilantro, chopped

1 tablespoon lemon juice

Directions:

- In a blender, add all ingredients and blend till smooth and frothy.
- Pour into 2 glasses and serve.

Healthy Herb Smoothie

Ingredients:

1 cup fresh carrot juice

2 cups frozen mango chunks

1 tablespoon fresh mint leaves

1 tablespoon fresh tarragon

1 tablespoon fresh basil

1 cup orange juice

Directions:

- In a blender, add all ingredients and blend till smooth and frothy.
- Pour into 2 glasses and serve.

Ginger Detox Smoothies

Ingredients:

1 cup almond milk

2 teaspoons ginger, chopped

½ cup blueberries

1 banana, sliced

2 cups kale leaves

1 tablespoon Chia seeds

2 tablespoons raw honey

1/8 teaspoon ground cinnamon

Directions:

- In a blender, add all ingredients and blend till smooth and frothy.
- Pour into 2 glasses and serve.

Smoothies Recipes

Strawberry Kale Smoothie

Ingredients

2 cups kale

1 cup strawberries, frozen

1 cup ice, crushed

6 ounces hemp milk

1 small banana

Direction

Add all ingredients in a blender and blend until smooth.

Apple Orange Smoothie

Ingredients

1 green apple, cored, chopped

1 large orange, peeled, chopped

6 ounces water, filtered

Freshly squeezed juice from 1 lime

2 cups kale

Direction

Add all ingredients in a blender and blend until smooth.

Kale Banana Smoothie

Ingredients

2 cups chopped kale

1 small banana

6 ounces hemp milk

1 cup pineapple, fresh, peeled, chopped

Direction

Add all ingredients in a blender and blend until smooth.

Cucumber Kale Smoothie

Ingredients

1 cup cucumber

3 cups kale, chopped

1 green apple, chopped

Freshly squeezed juice from ½ a lemon

6 ounces filtered water

¼ cup parsley

1 cup ice, crushed

1 pear

1 cup celery

Direction

Add all ingredients in a blender and blend until smooth.

Berry Spinach Smoothie

Ingredients

2 cups strawberries

2 cups raw spinach

1 banana

¼ cup carrot

½ cup blueberries

¾ cup water

¾ cup freshly squeezed orange juice

Direction

Add all ingredients in a blender and blend until smooth.

Pineapple Mango Smoothie

Ingredients

1 ½ cups mango

1 cup pineapple

2 cups raw spinach

1 cup coconut water

1 banana, chopped

Direction

Add mango, spinach, pineapple, banana, and coconut water in a blender. Blend until smooth.

Peach Kale Smoothie

Ingredients

1 peach

1 cup raw kale

2 apples, chopped

1 cup freshly squeezed orange juice

1 mango, pits removed, chopped

Direction

Add all ingredients in a blender and blend until smooth.

Avocado Banana Smoothie

Ingredients

1 avocado, peeled, pits removed

1 cup mango, cubed

2 cups raw kale

2 kiwi fruits, peeled

1 banana, chopped

1 cup filtered water

1 cup pineapple cubes

Direction

Add all ingredients in a blender and blend until smooth.

Grape Banana Smoothie

Ingredients

2 bananas, chopped

2 cups red grapes

2 cups fresh spinach

4 tbsp almond butter

2 cups almond milk, unsweetened

Direction

Add all ingredients in a blender and blend until smooth.

Pear Spinach Smoothie

Ingredients

4 pear

1 banana

2 cups fresh spinach

1 tsp cinnamon

2 cups unsweetened almond milk

Direction

Add all ingredients in a blender and blend until smooth.

Berry Smoothie

Ingredients

1 cup strawberries, fresh

1 cup blueberries, fresh

2 cups almond milk, unsweetened

½ cup almonds

Direction

Add all ingredients in a blender and blend until smooth.

Gingery Kale Smoothie

Ingredients

1 large handful raw kale

1" ginger, peeled

2 tbsp chia seeds

1 pure water

A wedge of lemon

1 handful spinach

Direction

Add all ingredients in a blender and blend until smooth.

Kale Banana Smoothie

Ingredients

1 cup coconut water

3 large handfuls of kale

2 tsp bee pollen

1 banana, chopped

Direction

Add all ingredients in a blender and blend until smooth.

Chard Mango Smoothie

Ingredients

1 bunch chard

2 mangoes, pits removed, chopped

1 pineapple, peeled, cubed

2 cups pure water

Direction

Add all ingredients in a blender and blend until smooth.

Grape Wheat Grass Smoothie

Ingredients

½ cup wheat grass, fresh

1 cup green grapes

½ cup water

½ cup pineapple

1 cup ice, crushed

Direction

Add all ingredients in a blender and blend until smooth.

Watermelon Lettuce Smoothie

Ingredients

¼ watermelon

1 mango, cubed

1 head butter lettuce

Direction

Add all ingredients in a blender and blend until smooth.

Pomegranate Berry

Ingredients

1 cup freshly made pomegranate juice

½ avocado, peeled

2 cups berries, mixed, frozen

1 cup water

Direction

Add all ingredients in a blender and blend until smooth.

Tropical Smoothie

Ingredients

1 cup raw kale

2 tbsp passion fruit, pureed

1 ½ cups pineapple chunks

1 ½ cups coconut milk, unsweetened

Direction

Add all ingredients in a blender and blend until smooth.

Tofu Strawberry Smoothie

Ingredients

½ cup strawberries

½ cup tofu

½ cup kale

½ banana

½ cup unsweetened almond milk

½ cup yogurt

Direction

Add all ingredients in a blender and blend until smooth.

Peach Arugula Smoothie

Ingredients

2 peaches

2 cups arugula

1 cup pure water

1 banana

Direction

Add all ingredients in a blender and blend until smooth.

Spiced Orange Smoothie

Ingredients

1 orange, peeled

½ tsp each; cinnamon and nutmeg

1 apple, chopped

Direction

Add all ingredients in a blender and blend until smooth.

Banana Smoothie

Ingredients

4 bananas, chopped

1 cup freshly squeezed orange juice

1 tbsp organic honey

2 cups organic yogurt

Direction

Add all ingredients in a blender and blend until smooth.

Fruity Smoothie

Ingredients

1 cup freshly squeezed orange juice

1 cup mango, cubed

1 cup pineapple, peeled, chopped

1 cup watermelon, cubed

1 cup strawberries, fresh

1 cup honeydew melon

½ cup crushed ice

Direction

Add all ingredients in a blender and blend until smooth.

Banana Berry Smoothie

Ingredients

2 bananas, chopped

1 ½ cups mixed berries

1 handful spinach

1 cup crushed ice

Direction

Add all ingredients in a blender and blend until smooth.

Easy Strawberry Lemonade

Strawberry lemonade with a healthy twist. Who doesn't like the refreshing flavors of summer? Try this in place of lunch and you've got a whole meal in one tall glass of delicious.

Ingredients

☐ 1 ½ cups cold water or sugar free sparkling water[*]

☐ 1 ½ cups ice chips

☐ 1 Tbsp. lemon juice (or ½ tsp. lemon extract)

☐ Strawberry meal replacement powder[†]

Grab It And Go Shake!

On the go and missing your daily nutritional needs? This is a quick and easy breakfast, lunch, or dinner for those days when meal time just isn't on the agenda.

Ingredients

☐ 1 cup ice chips

☐ Chocolate, Strawberry, or Vanilla meal replacement powder

☐ 16 ounces cold water

Orange Creamsicle Shake

Remember those pop-up ice cream treats you used to get off the friendly neighborhood ice cream truck? This tastes just as good and it's even healthy for you. For the nostalgic at heart.

Ingredients

☐ 1 ½ cups ice chips

☐ 1 cup water

☐ ½ tsp. Orange Extract

☐ 2 Tbsp. Orange juice (or more orange extract)

☐ Vanilla meal replacement powder

Strawberry Banana Smoothie

Strawberry and banana go together like bread and butter. Simple, basic, and Oh so good. For the days when the blender takes too long, just pop this into a blender bottle and presto!

Ingredients

☐ 1 cup ice chips

☐ 1 cup water

☐ 1 Tbsp. banana extract

☐ Strawberry meal replacement powder

Peppermint Patty Shake

Like its Peanuts cartoon namesake, this blender bottle drink has attitude. It's also got a refreshingly cool flavor.

Ingredients

☐ 1 tsp. Peppermint extract

☐ 1 cup water

☐ 1 cup ice chips

☐ Vanilla meal replacement powder

Chocolate Mint Shake

Like the Peppermint Patty, only with **Chocolate**. Who can resist that combination of yummy goodness?

Ingredients
- 1 tsp. Mint extract
- 1 cup water
- 1 cup ice chips
- Chocolate meal replacement powder

Grapefruit Surprise Shake

Don't knock it 'til you try it. The grapefruit juice adds a bit of tang to the sweet vanilla. Yummy especially on a hot summer afternoon.

Ingredients

- ¾ cup pure unsweetened Grapefruit juice
- 1 cup ice chips
- ¾ cup water
- Vanilla meal replacement powder
- Optional: grapefruit wedge for garnish

Restaurant Style Italian Soda

This blender bottle creation adds a bit of a fizzy burst. It's also very versatile in that you can add whatever flavor syrup your heart desires. Add a small dash of milk or cream and you've got your own fancy **Creamosa** as the French say.

Ingredients

☐ 1 ½ cups cold water

☐ 1 ½ cups ice chips

☐ Vanilla meal replacement powder

☐ ½ ounce flavored syrup of your choice

Root Beer Float

Yum. That's all one can say about this meal replacement version of a favorite summer treat. All you're missing is the ice cream...

Ingredients

☐ 1 ½ cups ice chips

☐ 1 ½ cups sparkling water

☐ 1 tsp. Root Beer extract

☐ Vanilla meal replacement powder

Blueberry Smoothie

This particular tasty treat is full of antioxidant and probiotic power. And it only takes a minute to prepare before you head out the door to that next activity.

Ingredients
- 1 cup milk
- 1 cup blueberry yogurt
- Vanilla meal replacement powder

Iced Coffee Shake

No need to go spend $5.00 on a cup of iced coffee at the nearest Starbucks. Just mix and drink, and you've got coffee and breakfast all in one handy blender bottle.

Ingredients
- 2 cups cold coffee[‡]
- 1 ½ cups ice chips
- Vanilla meal replacement powder

Iced Mocha Shake

Chocolate and coffee? Who could resist this delicious breakfast treat when it only takes a moment to mix and serve?

Ingredients

☐ 2 cups cold coffee

☐ 1 ½ cups ice chips

☐ Chocolate meal replacement powder

Maple Nut Shake

A nutty, warm flavor in a blender bottle for those who want a delicious and healthy Amaretto.

Ingredients
- ☐ 1 cup ice chips
- ☐ 16 ounces cold water
- ☐ ½ tsp. Maple extract
- ☐ ½ tsp. Almond extract
- ☐ Vanilla meal replacement powder

Almond Joy Shake

Wave goodbye to those rich, chocolate bar calories. This tasty treat means you can have dessert in place of dinner. You can even exchange the vanilla powder for chocolate and enjoy a heavenly flavor.

Ingredients
- 1 cup ice chips
- 16 ounces cold water
- ½ tsp. Almond extract
- ½ tsp. Coconut extract
- Vanilla meal replacement powder
- Optional coconut flakes for garnish

Banana Blast Smoothie

This treat is a blast to make and a blast to drink--just like it says. Just mix and go!

Ingredients
- 1 ½ cups water
- 1 cup ice chips
- ½ tsp. Banana extract
- Vanilla meal replacement powder

Chocolate Covered Banana Smoothie

You can **never** go wrong with Chocolate. Drink this in place of that Banana Ice Cream Sunday you were eyeing at the nearest ice cream parlor. Guilt free and delicious.

Ingredients
- 1 ½ cups water
- 1 cup ice chips
- ½ tsp. Almond extract
- ½ tsp. Banana extract
- Chocolate meal replacement powder

Chocolate Covered Cherries Smoothie

Chocolate covered cherries in a breakfast smoothie? You don't have to resist this healthy alternative treat.

Ingredients

☐ 1 ½ cups water

☐ 1 cup ice chips

☐ ½ tsp. Cherry extract

☐ Chocolate meal replacement powder

Conclusion

You still think that you can resist these green smoothies, making an impact on your life? Antioxidant, anti aging, beautifying, stress reducing, anti-depressant, skin cleansing and many other health benefits in just a single food drink which is known as a smoothie. We cannot neglect the importance of these green smoothies. We should make these smoothies a regular part of our diet. These smoothies are also famous because of their versatility. They can be made with different fruits and vegetables according to the need and taste. Green smoothies can be served any time. They can be served at breakfast, snacks and as a cooling and refreshing drink in the summer evening. I am sure now that you will never let all these benefits slip out of your hand.

www.ingramcontent.com/pod-product-compliance
Lightning Source LLC
Chambersburg PA
CBHW071438070526
44578CB00001B/133